2019 NORMAL PRESSURE HYDROCEPHALUS

This Dementia Strikes All Ages!

BELLER HEALTH

This book is dedicated to people diagnosed with normal pressure hydrocephalus, and their loved ones.

CONTENTS

ACKNOWLEDGMENTS

Thanks to the American Academy of Neurology, Atlanta Center for Medical Research, Alzheimer's Association, Alzheimer's Disease Center, Alzheimer's Disease Center of Northwestern University, Alzheimer's Foundation of America, American Academy of Neurology, Association for Frontotemporal Degeneration, Australia Neurological Research, CDC, Department of Health and Human Services, Duke University Medical Center, Emory Hospital, Harvard Medical School, Johns Hopkins Medicine, Mayo Clinic, National Aphasia Association, National Institute of Neurological Disorders and Strokes, National Library of Medicine, National Institute on Aging, National Institutes of Health, Prince of Wales Medical Research Institute, *PubMed*, Stanford Library School of Medicine, Stanford Medicine, UCSF Department of Neurology, UCSF Memory and Aging Center, University of Cambridge Neurology Unit, World Health Organization (WHO), *Journal of American Medical Association* (JAMA), and several other organizations that provided information used for this book. Thanks to everybody who assisted this book in a variety of important ways, and everybody at Beller Health Research Institute. To my editor, John Briggs, who helps me improve every book. To all sources and for the photos. Most of all, thanks to my wife, Nicola Beller.

FOREWORD

Before we begin *Normal Pressure Hydrocephalus,* let's review the series.

The *Dementia Risk Factors, Symptoms, Diagnosis, Stages, Treatment, Prevention* Series devotes a book to each dementia.

The series is organic, meaning it is an evolving work, and each book receives major annual updates. As science uncovers information, we add the important data in new editions.

The series also differentiates from most medical books because I write in everyday language. We might describe the writing goal in two ways:

1. Simplify the language where nonscientists and those outside the medical profession can comprehend.

2. Honor the science and facts, and the best scientists, researchers, and health professionals.

The series focuses a spotlight on dementias with no cure, nor accurate testing.

The books:

Dementia Risk Factors, Symptoms, Diagnosis, Stages, Treatment, Prevention, Prevention Series

Alzheimer's Risk Factors & Symptoms   boob

Behavioral Variant Frontotemporal Dementia (bvFTD)

Primary Progressive Aphasia (PPA)

Dementia with Lewy Bodies

Parkinson's disease

Huntington's Disease

Normal Pressure Hydrocephalus

Wernicke-Korsakoff Syndrome

LATE (Limbic-predominant age-related TDP-43 encephalopathy)

Among the worst news we can hear is that we or one of our loved ones has dementia. A killer disease with no cure pumps fear in the bravest souls.

I have witnessed how this medical condition destroys, not just the inflicted person, but their loved ones. Besides the patient, nobody suffers more than voluntary caregivers.

If I had a magic wand, I would wipe away the pain.

Instead, I study dementia year around to write and release annual updates.

Who is the reading audience?

The audience for this series falls in five categories.

Those diagnosed with dementia

If medical authorities diagnose you with dementia, my heart goes out to you. You're in for a long battle, and you want to slow the disease and extend the quality of life as long as possible.

Loved ones of those diagnosed

If your loved one has a dementia, he or she needs you. Depending on the type, the dementia causes behavioral problems, memory issues, motor decline, and other psychological and physical disorders. The learning curve is fast and changes as one moves from one stage to the next.

Medical professionals interested in a dementia overview

If you are a medical professional interested in a quick elementary lesson on Dementia, this is a good option.

Volunteer & professional caregivers

If you are a dementia caregiver, you are also in for a long difficult march. Dementia patients demand 24/7 care in later stages, requiring help to go to the bathroom, bathing, and with other basic daily functions.

Anybody interested in learning about a disease that strikes 1 of 6 Americans, and 1 of 3 seniors

This series is a good option for anybody who wants to gain a basic understanding of the 15 dementias.

While dementia is a scary disease, the series is not frightening. The books include the facts and science as they exist at the time of this writing.

As much as possible, we replace medical jargon with everyday language.

These books are a straightforward conversation warm and friendly.

Series First Lesson

Nothing I say or write should replace a competent doctor. Doctors, much like teachers, are part of a sacred profession.

While informal education is a lifetime pursuit, formal education is crucial. I detest the worst teachers, for they let down students and society, but I love and respect the best teachers, true pillars of society.

I also abhor incompetent, greedy doctors who let down their patients and society, but love and respect the best doctors. A wise course for the profession is to weed out incompetent, uncaring, corrupt doctors and medical professionals. The medical profession also should listen to and follow the best within their profession. The worst thing we can do is pretend all doctors (or any profession) are the same.

Nothing good I write about the medical profession includes incompetent, uncaring doctors, nurses, etc. And nothing bad I write about the medical profession includes the best.

Like when picking a school, you want one in the upper fifty percent, the same is true for medical facilities and doctors.

Although the series criticizes the profession when deserved, the first lesson in this series is *find a competent doctor.* If you have one, count your blessings. If you do not, find one.

A bad doctor is nothing more than a glorified idiot, a dangerous parasite who dishonors a noble profession. These people are smart enough to get through medical school, but greedy or otherwise flawed beyond redemption. A doctor who does not care for his or her patients is worse than worthless.

At some point, Big pharmaceuticals, Big Insurance, and their political puppets appointed doctors sanctioned drug dealers, the worse little or no better than those on the worst corners.

Find a competent, dedicated, caring, experienced, informed doctor who listens and respects your opinion, and writes prescriptions as a LAST RESORT.

I offer the same advice in all my health books. Without the right doctor, you are at the mercy of a profit-oriented health system that seldom puts the patient's interests first, second, or third.

However, nothing I say or write in these books or elsewhere means you should not see a doctor, should stop taking your medication, or otherwise undermine the medical profession's ability to diagnose and treat any medical symptoms you might experience.

What I want you to do is find a good doctor you trust with your life and ask him or her pointed questions concerning your health and any treatment they recommend.

How many dementias?

Not counting mixed dementia, there are sixteen primary dementia types:

1. Alzheimer's disease

Lewy body dementia

2. Dementia with Lewy bodies/DLB
3. Parkinson's disease dementia/PDD

Vascular dementia

4. Buerger's disease
5. Intestinal ischemic syndrome
6. Peripheral artery disease
7. Popliteal entrapment syndrome
8. Raynaud's phenomenon
9. Renal artery disease

Frontotemporal dementia (FTD)

10. Behavioral Variant Frontotemporal Dementia (bvFTD)
11. Primary Progressive Aphasia (PPA)

Other Dementias

12. Normal pressure hydrocephalus
13. Creutzfeldt-Jacob
14. Wernicke-Korsakoff
15. Huntington's disease
16. LATE (the newest dementia category)

17. *Mixed dementia

*Not a specific dementia, but a combination, mixed dementia is the seventeenth category important in any dementia discussion.

Any disease leading to dementia symptoms is a dementia type, but the 16 listed represent most cases.

The series teaches the basics for each dementia. You will learn certain patterns. While there are no known cures and these diseases are irreversible, we control many of the habits causing dementia.

While genetics, age, and luck play a role in dementia, like most diseases, most cases result from unhealthy habits.

We are not bashing those victimized by genetics and age, but most people own the ability to avoid or postpone dementia.

For instance, those who use tobacco and abuse alcohol skyrocket their chances of dementia, including Alzheimer's disease. You will learn how healthier habits increase your chances of never getting or slowing the dreadful disease.

Dementia is costly, deadly, and in most cases avoidable. The disease terrifies, but we are not helpless. A good defense is the best solution to any formidable offense, and in the fight to remain healthy, our best defense is developing a healthy lifestyle advocated in this book.

I do not promise you a miracle cure. Nor does financial gain guide my mission, but hopes of helping others.

I am a researcher, a nutritionist, and author, and witnessed Alzheimer's disease, and other dementias invade, destroy and kill loved ones. This series on dementia and Alzheimer's provides the average person around the world easy-to-learn books covering complicated medical subjects.

I will challenge the medical profession where necessary,

just as in my political books I criticize Congress and the United States government for their mistakes or shortcomings.

Not that I am smarter than the average doctor or politician, but I offer a perspective those inside the medical bubble cannot.

My brief career as a Congressional staffer taught me how difficult it is to maintain one's focus inside the bubble. Seeing the big picture is no less challenging inside the medical bubble motivated by profit.

Profiteers and those wanting to credit or discredit somebody funds too many studies to promote their own product or discredit somebody else's.

This book series holds no ulterior agenda. The small royalty fees are the only compensation. I have accepted no money from corporations to promote their product, nor do I have an ax to grind with anybody in the medical profession.

I hold a profound respect for ethical, competent, dedicated, and hardworking nurses, doctors, and other medical personnel. Nor is there anything wrong when medical-related businesses — including hospitals, pharmaceutical companies, and insurance companies — make a reasonable profit for worthy medical supplies and services. But, I detest those who inflate prices for desperate people, or are incompetent.

My goal is to provide you a simple, short, informational guide so you can understand the different dementias, their symptoms, and causes before it strikes your family. Dementia kills one out of every six Americans. No family, no matter how wealthy, no matter where located, no matter their race, no matter their educational level is immune from dementia.

I hope dementia never strikes your family.

Because dementia attacks one of six families, I wrote this series to help you prepare (as much as possible) for the 16 dementias.

As the series name suggests, each book covers symptoms, causes, diagnosis, treatment, stages, and prevention for dementia covered.

The text contains American and British English. I write in American English, but the research comes from the best studies worldwide. Therefore, quotes from British, Australian, and some other researchers are in British English. For integrity, I do not edit quotes.

Having explained the series, let's examine normal pressure hydrocephalus.

Chapter 1: NORMAL PRESSURE HYDROCEPHALUS

Let's begin our discussion by defining the word hydrocephalus. *Hydro[1]* means water and *cephalus[2]* implies head.

Although rarer than other dementias we've discussed, normal pressure hydrocephalus is yet another death-dealing disease. National Institute of Neurological Disorders and Stroke describe normal pressure hydrocephalus as one of the most mysterious dementias[3]:

> *Normal pressure hydrocephalus (NPH) is an abnormal buildup of cerebrospinal fluid (CSF) in the brain's ventricles, or cavities. It occurs if the normal flow of CSF throughout the brain and spinal cord is blocked in some way. This causes the ventricles to enlarge, putting pressure on the brain. Normal pressure hydrocephalus can occur in people of any age, but it is most common in the elderly. It may result from a subarachnoid hemorrhage, head trauma, infection, tumor, or complications of surgery. However, many people develop NPH even when none of these factors are present. In these cases the cause of the disorder is unknown.*

Since normal pressure hydrocephalus is a less prevalent

form of dementia, it's likely to be years before we figure out what these "unknown" causes might be.

Diagnosing normal pressure hydrocephalus is difficult because some symptoms overlap with Alzheimer's and other dementias. As every normal pressure hydrocephalus organization, researcher, or doctor attests; we need more funding for vital research.

How many Normal Pressure Hydrocephalus Types?

As with many dementias, normal pressure hydrocephalus has several subtypes. The disease's roots determine the normal pressure hydrocephalus subtypes.

- Acquired
- Congenital
- Compensated
- Communicating
- Non-communicating
- Communicating

Acquired Normal Pressure Hydrocephalus

Acquired normal pressure hydrocephalus occurs at or after birth.

Congenital Normal Pressure Hydrocephalus

Babies with congenital normal pressure hydrocephalus are born with the disease.

Compensated Normal Pressure Hydrocephalus

Compensated hydrocephalus is present at birth or in early childhood, but lingers, showing no symptoms into adulthood.

Communicating Normal Pressure Hydrocephalus

Medical authorities refer to hydrocephalus as communicating when cerebrospinal fluid flows uninterrupted through the brain's subarachnoid space and the ventricular system.

Non-Communicating Normal Pressure Hydrocephalus

Doctors refer to hydrocephalus as non-communicating when a tumor or something blocks or inhibits cerebrospinal fluid in the ventricular system.

We discuss each normal pressure hydrocephalus type in the next chapter on causes.

How Many People have Normal Pressure Hydrocephalus?

According to the Hydrocephalus Association, over 700,000 Americans suffer normal pressure hydrocephalus, but doctors often misdiagnose the symptoms as Parkinson's disease or Alzheimer's disease[4].

The number might be much higher.

According to the Cleveland Clinic[5], "as many as 10 percent of people with dementia attributed to other disorders may actually have NPH {normal pressure hydrocephalus)."

Who gets Normal Pressure Hydrocephalus?

Normal pressure hydrocephalus strikes most people over sixty[6], but attacks people all ages.

How Many Babies are Born with Normal Pressure Hydrocephalus?

Two of 1,000 babies are born with normal pressure hydrocephalus[7].

Is there a Cure for Normal Pressure Hydrocephalus?

Most dementias are incurable, but—if diagnosed early enough—the medical profession might reverse normal pressure hydrocephalus[8].

What are the Medical Costs for Normal Pressure Hydrocephalus?

Normal pressure hydrocephalus medical costs surpass $2 billion per year[9].

Chapter 2: WHAT CAUSES NORMAL PRESSURE HYDROCEPHALUS?

Researchers uncovered two pathways to normal pressure hydrocephalus:

1. Primary (idiopathic)

2. Secondary

Primary Normal Pressure Hydrocephalus

The cause remains unknown, but this form leads to gait problems, urinary incontinence, and dementia[10].

Secondary Normal Pressure Hydrocephalus

Tumors, subarachnoid hemorrhages, and head injuries are the primary causes of this version[11].

Chapter 3: HOW DO DOCTORS DIAGNOSE NORMAL PRESSURE HYDROCEPHALUS?

Almost 50 years after the original description of NPH, there still remain many unknowns, including its diagnostic criteria—
Hydrocephalus Association

Diagnosing normal pressure hydrocephalus frustrates health professionals, patients, and loved ones. One stands a far better chance of winning a coin toss than receiving an accurate normal pressure hydrocephalus diagnosis.

The Alzheimer's Association[12] laments over doctors misdiagnosing 80% of normal pressure hydrocephalus cases[13].

The Hydrocephalus Association[14] complains diagnosis criteria is inadequate and medical professionals too often misdiagnose normal pressure hydrocephalus for Parkinson's disease, Alzheimer's disease, or another neurological disorder[15].

If misdiagnosed for Alzheimer's, medical authorities consider the person incurable.

Early and correct diagnosis is crucial. One of the reversible dementias, an early and correct normal pressure hydrocephalus diagnosis is often the difference between life and death, tolerable and unbearable.

With no accurate, cheap, or quick test, how do doctors diagnose normal pressure hydrocephalus?

We refer to the under 20% when doctors make the correct diagnosis, not the 80% of the times they get it wrong.

To reach a correct diagnosis:

One, primary physicians and health professionals must receive better dementia training in all 16 primary dementias and their subtypes.

Two, primary physicians must refer patients to the right neurologists and others who specialist in normal pressure hydrocephalus.

Three, the specialists must:

- recognize the symptoms (Gait deterioration,
- run CAT scans and MRI's
- order cerebrospinal fluid tests
- order neuropsychological testing

If all this happens, and the neurologist ties the different signs together, he or she will make the correct diagnosis.

Let's view the normal pressure hydrocephalus diagnosis criteria.

Normal Pressure Hydrocephalus Diagnosis Criteria

A three-step process guides the diagnosis criteria[16].

1. **Clinical Examination**[17] confirms gait disturbance[18] and urinary urgency/incontinence[19], or dementia related cognitive decline[20].

2. **Brain imaging tests**[21] (CT scan[22] and/or MRI[23]) confirming hydrocephalus defined by the >30 Evans' ratio[24].

3. **Cerebrospinal fluid test**[25] predicts "shunt[26] responsiveness and/or determine shunt pressure include lumbar puncture, external lumbar drainage, measurement of CSF outflow resistance, intracranial pressure[27] (ICP) monitoring and isotopic cisternography[28]."

Tests Doctors use to Diagnose Normal Pressure Hydrocephalus?

According to the Cleveland Clinic, there are four primary tests to diagnose normal pressure hydrocephalus[29].

- Imaging tests
- Gait analysis
- Cerebrospinal fluid tests
- Neuropsychological testing

Imaging tests

- CT Scan

- MRI

MRI and CT scans support clinical diagnosis by confirming "enlarged lateral and third ventricles out of proportion to the cortical sulcal enlargement[30]."

Gait analysis

Medical authorities measure gait problems and compare the symptoms to those most prevalent in normal pressure hydrocephalus.

Medical authorities can tell much about our bones, muscles, and ligaments by how we walk.

Gait analysis measures two elements; the stance phase when both feet are secure to the ground and swing phase when one foot is off the ground.

Gait Measurements

To help distinguish between medical conditions such as Parkinson's disease and normal pressure hydrocephalus, the analysis covers a wide range of gait-related motion.

They examine cadence (rhythm), velocity, distance, autonomy (maximum walking time), routes, angles, width, momentum, posture, angles of feet, knees, legs, arms, upper body, neck, and head when walking.

Medical authorities also measure stop duration to determine gait severity and endurance.

Other Gait Measurements

- Gait phases
- Ground reaction forces
- How much electrical activity muscles produce
- Leg segment direction
- Maintaining gait over long time periods
- Long step length (distance between steps of both feet)
- Short step time

- Short step stride (distance between two successive steps by same foot)
- Swing time (time it takes each foot to lift the floor until touching again)
- Support time for each foot (when the heel touches the floor until lifting toes)
- Uneven terrain covered (height difference between drops and rises)

  Sources: *ScienceDirect*[31], *PubMed*[32], Forbes[33], Temple University School of Podiatric Medicine[34], Cleveland Clinic Lemer Research Institute[35], Johns Hopkins Medicine[36]

Specialists also watch for falls and tremors while walking. They measure everything conceivable because combinations of symptoms point medical professionals toward the correct diagnosis.

Specialists use two gait analysis types.

1. Model-based methods

2. Motion-based methods

Model-based methods

The model-based method uses math to measure the motion of one's body parts, including the arms, legs, head, neck, and waste through segmented images.

In 2007, Mark Nixon and Imed Bouchrika from the University of Southampton, UK developed the human model-based analysis[37].

> *We propose a new approach to extract human joints (vertex positions) using a model-based method. Motion templates describing the motion of the joints as derived by gait analysis, are parametrized using the elliptic Fourier descriptors. The heel strike data is exploited to reduce the dimensionality of the parametric models. People walk normal to the viewing plane, as major gait information is available in a sagittal view. The ankle, knee and hip joints are successfully extracted with high accuracy for indoor and outdoor data. In this way, we have established a baseline analysis which can be deployed in recognition, marker-less analysis and other areas.*

How accurate are the tests?

The authors concluded the tests "confirmed the robustness of the proposed method to recognize walking subjects with a correct classification rate[38].

Motion-based methods

Motion-based methods extract features from image sequences.

Hidden Morkov Models

A hidden Markov model uses new devices such as smart shoes to examine gait motions and phases by getting ground contact forces[39].

Gait Energy Image

In 2005, University of California researchers released a new spatio-temporal gait representation, which they named Gait Energy image to "characterize human walking properties for individual recognition by gait[40]."

Addressing inadequate training templates, the team also proposed[41]:

> *A novel approach for human recognition by combining statistical gait features from real and synthetic templates. We directly compute the real templates from training silhouette sequences, while we generate the synthetic templates from training sequences by simulating silhouette distortion. We use a statistical approach for learning effective features from real and synthetic templates. We compare the proposed GEI-based gait recognition approach with other gait recognition approaches on USF Human ID Database. Experimental results show that the proposed GEI is an effective and efficient gait representation for individual recognition, and the proposed approach achieves highly competitive performance with respect to the*

published gait recognition approaches.

Cerebrospinal fluid tests

Medical professionals use cerebrospinal fluid tests to predict shunt effectiveness in patients clinically diagnosed with normal pressure hydrocephalus.

Cerebrospinal fluid

A clear liquid, cerebrospinal fluid surrounding and protecting our central nervous system (brain and spinal cord). The U.S. National Library of Medicine explains how the central nervous system controls almost everything we consider us, and cerebrospinal fluid's role[42].

> *Your central nervous system controls and coordinates everything you do including, muscle movement, organ function, and even complex thinking and planning. CSF (cerebrospinal fluid) helps protect this system by acting like a cushion against sudden impact or injury to the brain or spinal cord. CSF also removes waste products from the brain and helps your central nervous system work properly.*

Medical authorities favor the lumbar puncture (spinal tap) to test cerebrospinal fluid, but there are other options such as fluoroscopy, cisternal puncture, and ventricular puncture[43].

Medical professionals check to see if there is too much cerebrospinal fluid surrounding and placing pressure on the brain.

The test is important for two reasons:

1. To diagnose normal pressure hydrocephalus.
2. To predict how effective a ventriculoperitoneal shunt might be in treating cerebrospinal fluid

pressure.

"When spinal fluid builds up in the ventricles, it causes them to enlarge and stretch the brain tissue," explained NYU Langone Health. "This can lead to problems with walking, cognitive impairment—such as memory problems and dementia—and diminished bladder control[44]."

Neuropsychological testing

Many gait analysis commercial wearable sensors are on the market today. These each gather gait analysis for runners, athletes, and for those suffering gait-related medical problems.

The Department of Neurosurgery, University of Cambridge School of Clinical Medicine described neuropsychological testing's importance[45].

> *Clinical neuropsychology provides a means of determining a cognitive profile for NPH, assisting in differential diagnosis, tracking the disorder's progression and assessing the efficacy of treatment. This article will review possible applications of clinical neuropsychology and propose a clinical assessment protocol for NPH.*

Chapter 4: TREATMENT FOR NORMAL PRESSURE HYDROCEPHALUS

Medical professionals can treat normal pressure hydrocephalus in early stages, but the success rate drops as the medical condition progresses[46].

According to the Hydrocephalus Association, only one of five people with normal pressure hydrocephalus receive correct treatment[47].

This is tragic considering normal pressure hydrocephalus is one of the few dementias doctors can reverse.

A key to reversal is early diagnosis, but officials misdiagnose 80% of cases, and fail to treat 4 of 5 normal pressure hydrocephalus sufferers.

Once again, I stress the need for more research funds for normal pressure hydrocephalus.

Pacific Adult Hydrocephalus Center[48] suggests two treatment forms[49].

1. Lumbar puncture

2. Ventriculoperitoneal shunt

Lumbar Puncture (Spinal Tap)

The lumbar puncture, also known as spinal tap, helps doctors diagnose normal pressure hydrocephalus[50], but also is one of two primary treatments (the other is the ventriculoperitoneal shunt).

If the procedure provides relief, this indicates normal pressure hydrocephalus. Besides helping diagnose normal pressure hydrocephalus, medical professionals use the lumbar puncture to provide pain relief.

A neurosurgeon performs a lumbar puncture in the lower back in the lumbar area, inserting a needle between the vertebrae to collect a cerebrospinal fluid sample[51].

Although the cerebrospinal fluid protects the brain and spinal cord, an excess amount places pressure on the brain and causes the symptoms associated with normal pressure hydrocephalus[52].

The lumbar puncture measures cerebrospinal fluid pressure[53].

Lumbar Puncture Risk Factors

According to the Mayo Clinic, the procedure poses the following risk factors[54]:

- Back pain (pain might carry to back of legs)
- Bleeding (rare)
- Brainstem herniation (when a brain tumor is present)
- Headaches (up to 25 percent)

Ventriculoperitoneal Shunt

Ventriculoperitoneal shunts are the primary form of treating normal pressure hydrocephalus.

Neurosurgeons implant ventriculoperitoneal shunts to drain excess cerebrospinal fluid from the brain. The shunt comes in three parts[55].

- The ventricular catheter
- A valve regulating cerebrospinal fluid
- A catheter running into the abdominal space

The neurosurgeon scalps an incision in the back of head and drills a hole into the skull[56]. Inside the enlarged ventricle, the neurosurgeon passes the catheter through the brain.

A neurosurgeon inserts a shunt valve through an incision behind the ear and attaches the ventricular catheter[57].

A surgeon team makes a third incision in the belly and form a tunnel from the ear, down the chest to the abdominal. The system pumps excess cerebrospinal fluid from the brain to the belly[58], which absorbs and disperses the excess fluid.

The procedure helps many with the gait and continence problems, but Johns Hopkins Medicine warns shunts do not relieve dementia symptoms[59].

"Most types of dementia (e.g. Alzheimer's dementia) cannot be cured, but only temporized," according to Pacific Adult Hydrocephalus Center. "There are very few types of reversible dementia–one of these is Normal Pressure Hydrocephalus. Normal pressure hydrocephalus is a rare dementia the medical profession can sometimes reverse. If you show symptoms, see a doctor (neurologist). The sooner you do, the greater chance of preventing the medical condition from destroying your life and leading to premature death."

If you have normal pressure hydrocephalus symptoms, please see a doctor (neurologist) as soon as possible.

Chapter 5: STAGES & SYMPTOMS FOR NORMAL PRESSURE HYDROCEPHALUS

Normal pressure hydrocephalus lacks the stages established for Alzheimer's and most dementias because it lags in research. Also, unlike other dementias, normal pressure hydrocephalus is often reversible.

We know the symptoms and, if untreated, grow more severe. Untreated or maltreated, normal pressure hydrocephalus causes premature death like most dementias.

What are symptoms of normal pressure hydrocephalus?

The symptoms and progression differ from patient-to-patient, but below are common.

- Attention deficit[60]
- Bradyphrenia[61] (rigidity, weakness, tremors)
- Impaired thinking skills[62]
- Inability to control the bladder[63]
- Irritability[64]
- Memory loss[65]
- Walking difficulty[66]
- Injury from fall[67]

Normal pressure hydrocephalus requires more studies, but this is one form of dementia that neurosurgeons can reduce through surgery if caught soon enough[68]. Unless examined by a neurosurgeon, doctors often misdiagnose normal pressure hydrocephalus.

Children and adults experience different normal pressure hydrocephalus. Because their fibrous joints connecting bones in the skull are unclosed, children can better adapt to cerebrospinal fluid buildup than adults.

Most Obvious Normal Pressure Hydrocephalus Symptoms for Children

While children better adapt to the cerebrospinal fluid buildup, their heads grow unusually large.

Other Normal Pressure Hydrocephalus Symptoms for Children

- Head soft spot bulges
- Skull bone gaps (split sutures)
- Irritability
- Seizures
- Sleepy
- Sun setting (Downward eyes)
- Swollen veins
- Vomiting

Normal Pressure Hydrocephalus Symptoms for Older Children & Adults

As we age, the more our heads and brains set, so the initial symptoms are more severe for older children and adults.

Most older children and adults with normal pressure hydrocephalus first suffer headaches.

Cerebrospinal fluid buildup puts pressure on the brain, causing headaches.

Other Normal Pressure Hydrocephalus Symptoms for Older Children & Adults

While they vary from one person to the next, symptoms for adults and older children include suffer a variety of physical, cognitive, and urinary issues.

- Blurred vision
- Dementia
- Depression
- Double vision
- Cognitive decline
- Drowsy
- Gait decline
- Impaired coordination
- Irritable
- Lethargic
- Memory loss
- Nausea
- Poor balance

- Sun setting
- Urinary incontinence
- Vomiting

Parkinson's disease and Creutzfeldt-Jakob share a long list of symptoms, explaining why doctors often misdiagnose normal pressure hydrocephalus.

Symptoms Sources: American Association of Neurological Surgeons[69], Joseph H. Piatt Jr., MD[70], Child Neurology Foundation[71], Harvard Medical School[72], National Organization of Rare Disorders[73] (NORD), Johns Hopkins Medicine[74], National Health Service[75] (NHS),

Chapter 6: RISK FACTORS FOR NORMAL PRESSURE HYDROCEPHALUS

What are risk factors for normal pressure hydrocephalus?

We need more research to confirm, but the disease appears to result from brain disorders[76]:

- Age 60 or over[77]
- Brain infections[78]
- Brain surgery history[79]
- Brain tumors[80]
- Head injuries[81]
- Hemorrhages[82]
- Inflammation[83]

I suspect several indirect risk factors, including any unhealthy habits causing high blood pressure, high cholesterol, diabetes, and other medical conditions increasing all dementia type risks.

In the bonus section on how to possibly prevent or slow normal pressure hydrocephalus and other dementias, we discuss how to maximize our defense against any disease.

We'll update this section when new studies confirm other risk factors.

We need more research!

CHAPTER 7: BONUS SECTION

Starter To-do List for Somebody and Family once Diagnosed with Dementia.

The person with dementia, loved ones, and family must address several matters early in the disease, including:

- **Care:** Family, loved ones, and dementia patient must make difficult decisions concerning if somebody can become the primary volunteer caregiver. While dementia patients do not require 24/7 care in the early stage, it becomes necessary in middle to late stages.

- **Financial decisions:** There are significant financial decisions to make, and earlier the better. Such a disease becomes a hardship for not only the patient but also their family. The demands, financial and otherwise, on voluntary caregivers often is devastating. Make difficult financial decisions early.

- **Living Quarters:** While most dementia patients maintain independence in stage one, at some point they require help with daily tasks. Will somebody move in with her or him? Does the patient move in with somebody else? Will it become necessary for him or her to move into an assisted living community in later stages?

- **Living Will**: It is crucial to document dementia patient's wishes while he or she maintains their facilities to make such decisions.

- **Power of Attorney**: It is important to establish a Power of Attorney to empower a trusted loved one to make medical and financial decisions when a patient becomes incapable.

Above is an incomplete list. Once diagnosed, both the person diagnosed and loved ones must unite and build your own to-do list.

Possible Ways To Prevent Or Slow Normal Pressure Hydrocephalus & The Other 15 Dementias

Besides how cruel dementia is, the worst aspect might be the disease is incurable. Therefore, it is crucial we build our own defense system and do our best to prevent or slow these and other devastating diseases.

We've developed a 12-point plan to reduce your risks of getting, or slowing if you already have one of the 16 dementias.

The habits and principles discussed in this chapter not only reduce your chances of getting or increase your chances of fighting dementia, but also provide the tools for us to be our healthiest, happiest, and most productive selves.

I discuss the principles in greater detail in Be the Best You!

12-Point Plan to become Your Healthiest, Happiest, & Most Productive, & Possibly Prevent or Slow Normal Pressure Hydrocephalus & other Dementias

1. Avoid or limit drinking to 1 drink per day (female adults) or 2 (male adults).
2. Do not smoke or otherwise use tobacco products.
3. Eat a balanced, whole food diet (avoiding processed food).
4. Exercise 4-7 times per week, manage weight and keep within healthy margins. Avoid belly fat.
5. Socialize and remain active.
6. Read and otherwise exercise your mind.
7. Follow the Golden Rule, avoid negativity, shine a light.
8. Manage and control blood pressure, blood sugar, & cholesterol.
9. Avoid or treat stress, anxiety, and depression.
10. Don't demand or expect prescription drugs for every symptom. Ask questions about side effects.
11. Find legitimate reasons to laugh more than the average person.
12. Remain hydrated and avoid sugary drinks.

Above is the short list, but you'll gain incredible benefits if you follow those 12 suggestions.

Balanced, whole food diet

Few things like health and exercise predict one's health. No matter one's gender, race, nation, demographics, if all we know is their diet and amount of exercise, we can predict if they are healthy or unhealthy.

If we know somebody smokes, we can predict health issues and symptoms they might experience based on how much tobacco they consume.

If somebody is obese, we can predict associated health issues like high blood pressure, diabetes, and several cardiovascular issues.

In contrast, if a doctor knows somebody eats a balanced whole food diet and exercises 30-60 minutes five to seven times per week, he or she knows this person has reduced their risks and increased their ability to fight or slow dementia.

The food you eat can be either the safest and most powerful form of medicine or the slowest form of poison. — Dr. Ann Wigmore

Is your diet a "powerful form of medicine" or a recipe to tedious suicide?

Balanced whole foods including Omega-3, vegetables, fruits, beans, nuts, berries (blueberries), carotenoids, genistein, tea (green), coffee (black), spinach, unfried fish (salmon), flax seeds, chia seeds, kale, whole grains, and resveratrol are among the specific foods that lower risk of dementia.

A *PubMed* study found coconut oil, fresh herbs and spices, red wine, and olive oil reduce dementia's risk[84].

The table below is incomplete but provides the best evidence current science provides. I divided the table into three categories: 1) Bad foods that cause neurogeneration; 2) Foods that require more studies. 3) Good foods providing neuroprotection.

Bad Foods/Need more Studies/Good Foods

The table below shows confirmed bad foods on the left, and science-backed good foods on the right. In the middle are foods requiring more studies, although the arrows point towards the direction preliminary studies show.

Bad foods	Need more studies	Good foods
Dairy	MUFA→	Omega-3
High fructose corn syrup	←PUFA	Fresh Vegetables
White sugar	←Saturated Fat	Fresh Fruits
Trans fat	Vitamin C→	Nuts (Walnuts, Cashews, Macadamia)
	Vitamin D→	
	Vitamin E →	
	Riboflavin→	Berries (Blueberries)
	←Carbohydrates	
	←Meat	Olive Oil
	Coconut Oil→	

		Fresh herbs & spices
		Unfried fish
		(Wild caught Salmon)
		Tea
		Coffee
		Resveratrol
		Carotenoids
		Genistein

We need more studies to expand the list, but this provides a good roadmap to an anti-dementia diet. Include as many of the proven neuroprotection foods — herbs, spices, teas, coffee, and supplements — in your diet as possible.

A whole food diet includes:

- Whole grains (no white or processed flour!)
- Vegetables
- Fruit
- Salmon (Free caught fish)
- Blueberries

- Green tea (or other unsweetened teas)
- Coffee (unsweetened)

Supplements

- Resveratrol

Exercise

Physical activity promotes cardiovascular health, enhances cognitive skills, and improves one's longevity chances.

Humans build strength through exercise. Muscles without exercise turn to fat, which we must carry around like a bowling ball bag (or two or three). As we become weaker, we must carry larger and larger loads (us). This increases our chances of:

- Physical injury
- Obesity
- High blood pressure
- Cardiovascular disease
- Strokes
- Dementia (including LATE)
- Parkinson's disease
- Other diseases and medical conditions

Exercising reduces the risks for all diseases and medical conditions listed. Exercise four to seven times per week.

The NIH's *Physical Activity Guidelines for Americans* summarizes the human costs.

> *About $117 billion in annual health care costs and about 10 percent of premature mortality are associated with inadequate physical activity (not meeting the aerobic key guidelines).*

Health Benefits from Exercising

- Better sleep
- Congestive heart failure
- Cognitive function benefits
- Decrease cancer risks
- Decrease early mortality risk
- **Decrease dementia risk**
- Decrease diabetes risk
- Decrease stress
- Fewer fall-related injuries
- Greater physical ability and well-being
- Improves quality of life
- Improves physical ability
- Lessons cancer risks (for several types)
- Lower blood pressure
- Promotes bone health
- Promotes brain health
- Reduces anxiety
- Reduces depression
- Reduces stroke risk
- Weight control

> **Sources**: Mayo Clinic[85], CDC[86], "Physical Activity Guidelines for Americans[87], university of Alberta[88], Department of Biomedical Sciences, University of Missouri[89], Institute for Research in Extramural Medicine, VU University Medical Center[90], Department of Human Movement and Exercise Science, The University of Western Australia[91]

A study released February 2019 in *Neurology* tested how

exercise affects dementia risk. The researchers concluded: "midlife cognitive and physical activities are independently associated with reduced risk of dementia and dementia subtypes. The results indicate that these midlife activities may have a role in preserving cognitive health in old age[92]."

Another study released in the *Journal of Clinical Pathology* studied 7501 senior citizens over nine years. "Regular exercise was associated with decreased risk of dementia," said lead author Zi Zhou. "Policy-makers should develop effective public health programs and build exercise-friendly environments for the general public[93]."

A longitudinal population study followed 1,462 women over 42 years to measure physical activity's relation to dementia and found those who exercised lowered their dementia risks by 88 percent. Study first author Helena Hörder, professor, Department of Psychiatry and Neurochemistry, University of Gothenburg in Sweden explained the results.

"Our findings indicate that high cardiovascular fitness in midlife is associated with decreased risk of dementia," said Hörder. "Improved cardiovascular fitness in midlife might be a modifiable factor to delay or prevent dementia[94]."

Did the results surprise the researchers?

"I was not surprised that there was an association," said Hörder. "but I was surprised that it was such a strong association between the group with highest fitness and decreased dementia risk[95]."

A University of Cambridge study released in *Lancelot* engaged a 10-year study and determined exercise can cut dementia risks by a third[96]. Professor Carol Brayne, Cambridge Institute of Public Health, University of Cambridge, served as the lead author. "Although there is no single way to prevent dementia, we may reduce our risk of developing dementia at older ages. We know what many of these factors are, and that they are often linked," said Brayne. "Simply tackling physical inactivity, for example, will reduce levels of obesity, hypertension and diabetes, and prevent some people from developing dementia and a healthier old age in general–it's a win-win situation."

Pointers

The National Institute of Health's "Physical Activity Guidelines for Americans" recommend the following[97]:

- "Move more, sit less"
- Any physical activity is better than none
- Exercise a minimum of 2 ½ hours per week of moderate-intensity exercise, or 1 hour and 14 minutes of vigorous-intensity exercises
- Gain additional benefits by going beyond the minimum amount
- Spread exercise across the week (avoid consecutive off days)
- Do resistance exercises for muscle-building 2-4 days per week

If you suffer a chronic medical condition limiting your physical ability, do what you can. No matter our physical condition, each of us must push ourselves to do what we can and keep increasing our potential. As professor Brayne said, exercise is a "win-win situation." The more we exercise, the stronger we become, and nature keeps raising the bar.

As the NIH suggests, "move more, sit less." Did you know sitting too much can be deadly? Modern humans sit too much, which is why sitting earns its own section.

The question is not if but how we should exercise. Let's review several great options.

Walking

Our ancestors walked wherever they went. There were no cars, subways, elevators, escalators, sitting-jobs, and other luxuries costing us our necessary steps per day.

Then came the horse and buggy, trains, early elevators, and by 1913 the Model T. From there, humans have been working night and day to avoid walking.

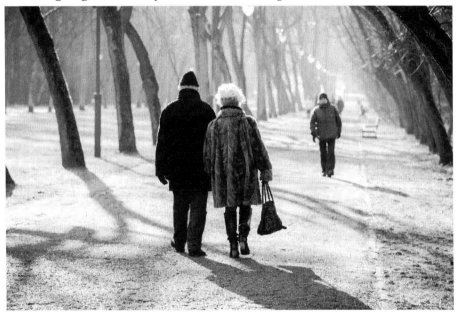

Go for walks!

A *Annals of Internal Medicine* study found who walked[98] three or more times per week decreased their dementia risk by 38% compared to those who did not exercise[99].

Another study published in Journal of Neurology formed four groups:

1. Group One ate a DASH[100] diet (Dietary Approaches to Stop Hypertension).

2. Group Two exercise, but received no special diet instruction. Supervised exercise included 10 minutes warming up and 35 minutes walking.
3. Group Three adopted the DASH diet and took part in the walking program.
4. The fourth group received a thirty-minute cardiovascular instruction over the phone, but did not exercise or change their diets.

Study lead author James Blumenthal, Duke University clinical psychologist explained their findings. "Our operating model was that by improving cardiovascular risk, you're also improving neurocognitive functioning," said Blumenthal. "You're improving brain health at the same time as improving heart health."

The researchers found Group Three, those who adopted the Dash diet and took part in the exercise group achieved the greatest benefits. Next best, Group Two that participated in the exercise program with no diet changes.

Richard Isaacson, Director of Alzheimer's Prevention Clinic[101], Weill Cornell Medicine[102], weighed in on the study.

"The results showed that controlled aerobic activity within a very short period of time can have a significant impact on the part of the brain that keeps people taking care of themselves, paying their bills and the like," said Isaacson. "Not only can you improve, but you can improve within six months!"

What we do today affects our future physical and cognitive health. "You can do something today for a better brain tomorrow," said Isaacson.

Walk in nature, breathe fresh air, enjoy nature, absorb some vitamin D, and reduce your risks for dementia and other life-threatening diseases. Walk several times per week and achieve a healthier, happier version of you.

Running

If you are healthy enough, running pumps the heart, clears the lungs, and strengthens our muscles and internal organs.

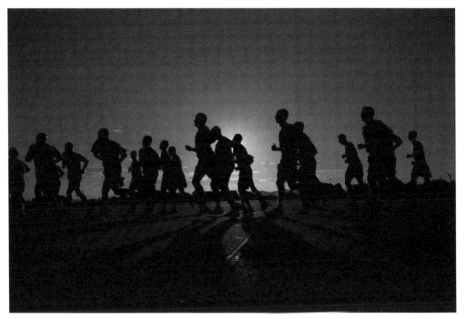

Run by yourself or with others!

You can run by yourself, with a partner, or group, but do so 3-5 times per week.

Remember to stretch before and after. Dress in the right running shoes and apparel. Take water.

A *Journal of Alzheimer's Disease* study followed 154,000 runners and walkers for 11 years. The researchers concluded those who run 7.7-15.3 miles per week reduced dementia risks by 25%, while those who ran 15 miles or more per week reduced risks by 40 percent[103].

If you are able, run. Running improves your physical and cognitive health, extends your quality-of-life.

Hiking

Hiking is a terrific option to get exercise and explore nature. Avoid danger, and consult a doctor if you have any health issues, but there are dozens of hiking options within a short driving distance of most everywhere.

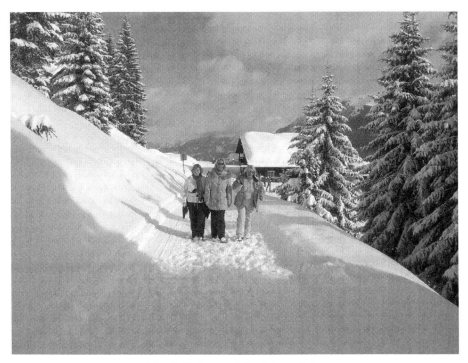

Go hiking with friends!

Whatever hiking you can handle, go for it!

Swimming

If available, swimming is a fantastic regular exercise.

If you do not have another option, become a member of the YMCA or another local club, and go 5-7 days per week. The swimming will strengthen your body and provide endless hours of fun.

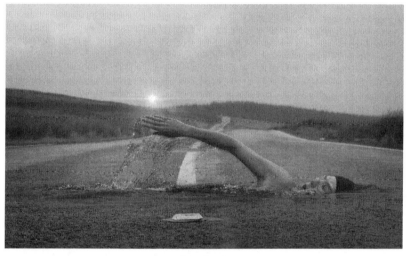

Swim!

I chose physical activities a person can do alone or with another person.

Tennis and other sports are great but require partners. If you choose such a sport, set up backup partners for when your partner is sick, out of town, etc.

Avoid depression

As we covered in early chapters, research connects depression to dementia, but researchers are uncertain whether as a cause or symptom.

Either way, we need to reduce depression. It disrupts our cognitive health and makes us more susceptible to dozens of medical conditions.

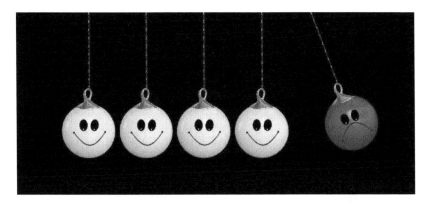

Keep the smile and stop depression!

Researchers from the Department of Neurology, Genetics Program, Boston University designed a "cross-sectional, family-based, case-control" study including 1,953 people with Alzheimer's disease and 2,093 of their relatives who did not have Alzheimer's. Robert C. Green[104], MD, MPH, Harvard Medical School served as the project's lead author.

"Depression symptoms before the onset of AD are associated with the development of AD, even in families where first depression symptoms occurred more than 25 years before the onset of AD," said Green. "These data suggest that depression symptoms are a risk factor for later development of AD[105].

A National Institute of Health sponsored longitudinal study followed 1,239 older people for 24.7 years to determine if depression increased dementia risk. "Our findings support the hypothesis that depression is a risk factor for dementia and suggest that recurrent depression is particularly pernicious," said the researchers. "Preventing the recurrence of depression in older adults may prevent or delay the onset of dementia[106]."

As covered in the risk factors section, we need more studies to determine the exact link. Depression may cause dementia, or it might be an early symptom. Whatever the relationship to dementia, depression is torturous at the moment, and creates long-term health risks.

Depression demands diligence. Help yourself but seek help if required. Navigate to places and people who make you happy, and when possible avoid people and places that depress and make you sad.

People and places are not the only causes of depression. There are many physical, hormonal, and neurological possibilities.

As covered in earlier chapters, we must view depression and mental illnesses for the serious medical condition they are. Seek professional help if required. There is no more shame in seeking medical help for emotional or cognitive troubles than for a broken bone or flu symptoms.

Don't smoke

Do not smoke!

Among the zillion reasons not to smoke is it increases your risk 100% responsible for some vascular dementias, and directly or indirectly increases risk for all 16 dementias.

Researchers from the Centre for Mental Health Research, Australian National University conducted a meta-analysis study of 19 prospective studies. The research team concluded: "elderly smokers have increased risks of dementia and cognitive decline[107]."

A team of Finland researchers examined a "prospective data from a multiethnic population-based cohort," including 21,123 people to determine the smoking's impact on dementia. In their conclusions, the team said: "heavy smoking in midlife was associated with a greater than 100% increase in risk of dementia, AD, and VaD more than 2 decades later. These results suggest that the brain is not immune to long-term consequences of heavy smoking[108]."

Several other studies also link smoking to dementia. While we need more studies to determine if smoking causes dementia, we know it causes several medical conditions that increase one's dementia risk.

If you don't smoke, don't start. If you smoke, quit. There is not one good reason to consume tobacco products, but a million sound reasons not to avoid or kick the nasty habit.

More Reasons You Should Not Smoke or Use Tobacco Products

- Cigarettes include over 7,000 chemicals, over 70

linked to cancer

- Each day, over 3,200 children under 18 light their first cigarette
- Each year, over 41,000 Americans die from second-hand smoke.
- Annual tobacco costs Americans $332 billion in lost productivity and health care costs
- Over 16 million Americans live with tobacco-caused medical conditions
- Science links tobacco to bronchitis, cancer (several types), chronic airway obstruction, emphysema, erectile dysfunction, eye diseases, immune system deterioration, strokes, rheumatoid arthritis, tuberculosis, and type-2 diabetes
- Tobacco-related illness costs Americans $170 billion each year
- Tobacco kills one of five people in the United States
- Tobacco kills over 7 million people worldwide each year
- Tobacco kills almost 500,000 Americans each year
- Tobacco use robs ten years from the average smoker's life
- The leading cause of preventable deaths is tobacco in the United States and World

Sources: American Lung Association[109], CDC[110], WHO[111], New England Journal of Medicine[112], Federal Trade Commission[113], Department of Neurology, University Hospital School of Medicine[114], Comprehensive Cardiovascular Center, Saint Vincent Catholic Medical Centers of New York[115], FDA/CDC Joint Study[116]

Avoid anxiety

As with depression, scientists do not know if anxiety is a cause or a symptom, but either way you should take steps to avoid or limit anxiety.

According to the American Psychological Association[117], Anxiety is "an emotion characterized by feelings of tension, worried thoughts and physical changes like increased blood pressure[118]."

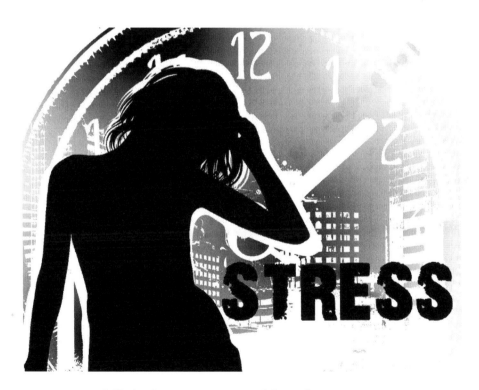

Minimize stress to avoid anxiety.

Premature Aging

Researchers from Brigham and Women's Hospital studied anxiety's affect the brain. "Many people wonder about whether—and how—stress can make us age faster," said lead author Olivia Okereke. "So, this study is notable for showing a connection between a common form of psychological stress— phobic anxiety—and a plausible mechanism for premature aging."

Funded in part by Harvard Medical, Okereke and the other researchers viewed blood samples from 5,243 women age 42-69 in a nurse's health study. Okereke and the team found anxiety caused the brain to premature age six years[119].

If stress causes premature brain aging and shortens telomeres, are there positive steps to accomplish the opposite?

According to UCSF[120], we can reduce stress, opening more blood flow to the brain, and lengthen our minimize aging through health habits advocated in this chapter. Researchers from UCSF and the Preventive Medicine Research Institute[121]."

Founder and president of the Preventive Medicine Research Institute, Dean Ornish[122], MD, UCSF clinical professor of medicine spoke for the group. "Our genes, and our telomeres, are not necessarily our fate," said Ornish. "So often people think 'Oh, I have bad genes, there's nothing I can do about it. But these findings indicate that telomeres may lengthen to the degree that people change how they live. Research indicates that longer telomeres are associated with fewer illnesses and longer life[123]."

A Canadian study published in the American Journal of Geriatric Psychiatry[124] gauged whether anxiety increases Alzheimer's and dementia symptoms. The research team reviewed cognitive changes every six months and found mild anxiety increased Alzheimer's risks by 33%, moderate anxiety by 78%, and severe anxiety by 135% or more[125].

Another study released in *Frontiers in Neuroscience*[126] followed 5,230 people for ten years, checking them every two years to determine anxiety's relation to dementia. Their findings backed other studies concluding anxiety increases dementia risks[127].

A *JAMA Psychiatry*[128] study focused 54 months on multi-center facilities treating Alzheimer's testing anxiety's relationship to cognitive decline in AD patients.

Lead author Robert Pietrzak[129], PhD, MPH, Associate Professor of Psychiatry and Public Health, U.S. Department of Veterans Affairs National Center for PTSD[130] summarized their findings.

"The results of our study suggest that among older adults with a positive beta-amyloid scan, those with elevated anxiety symptoms show a more rapid decline in global cognition, verbal memory, language, and executive function over a 54-month period," said Pietrzak. "This suggests that increased levels of anxiety increase the development of the symptoms of Alzheimer's disease. Thus, assessment, monitoring, and treatment of such symptoms, even subclinical levels, may help inform risk stratification and management of preclinical and prodromal phases of Alzheimer's disease[131]."

Besides anxiety increasing dementia risk, Harvard Medical School[132] warns several anxiety medications increase dementia risk[133].

Benzodiazepines Prescribed for Anxiety that Increase Dementia Risks

- alprazolam (Xanax)
- chlordiazepoxide (Librium)
- clonazepam (Klonopin)
- clorazepate (Tranxene)
- diazepam (Valium)
- flurazepam (Dalmane)
- lorazepam (Ativan)
- oxazepam (Serax)
- paroxetine (Paxil)

National Health Service[134] in Great Britain suggests anxiety and depressions role in dementia risks might be indirect, hypothesizing if one suffers anxiety, stress, or depression, they are less likely to socialize[135] (important in avoiding dementia).

Either way, we should avoid anxiety.

Anxiety and depression also cause high blood pressure and other medical conditions increasing dementia risks, so at a minimum there is an indirect link.

To reach anxiety, one must suffer stress first. Minimize stress and avoid anxiety.

Stop raging at every irresponsible driver. Do not

torture yourself over things that might happen when you know such worries almost come true. Do not confront every person who deserves a tongue-lashing.

I am not suggesting you become a pushover but knowing when to fight and when not to is an art one must learn to avoid stress.

Stress kills. Do not allow it to kill you!

Don't abuse alcohol

If you care about your health, you have two alcohol choices:

1. Do not drink alcohol.
2. Do not abuse alcohol.

This is not a goody-goody message, but a legitimate health risk warning.

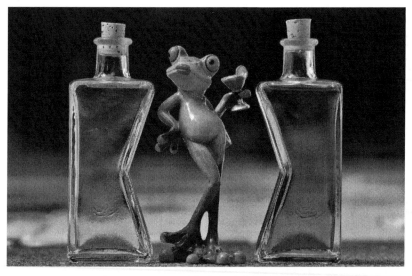

Do not exceed drinking limits!

The limit for women is one beer, a glass of wine, or cocktail per day, no exceptions.

Medical authorities set the limit for men to two beers, glasses of wine, or cocktails, no exceptions.

The rules include occasional drinkers. It does not matter if you limit drinking to once per week, month, or year, do not exceed the daily limit!

Does Alcohol Increase Dementia Risks?

French researchers released a study in Lancet linking alcohol use to an increased dementia risk. The team analyzed 31 million people released from national-wide French hospitals. "Alcohol use disorders were a major risk factor for onset of all types of dementia, and especially early-onset dementia[136]." Heavy drinkers were three times more likely to get dementia than those who did not abuse alcohol. They also found fifty percent of early-onset dementia was alcohol-related.

While the research was exclusive to the French population, 31 million people is a large sample size.

A group of Canadian researchers examined 28 systematic review published in PsycINFO, Embase, and Medline between 2000 and 2017 and concluded: "Heavy alcohol use was associated with changes in brain structures, cognitive impairments, and an increased risk of all types of dementia[137]."

Avoid the madness of alcohol abuse!

Don't demand or expect prescription drugs for every symptom. Ask questions about side effects

Not only can prescription drugs increase one's dementia risks, but the list of other potential side effects are far greater than the benefits.

Anybody who watches television in the United States if forgiven if their heads spin when the drug commercials spend most the commercial listing the potential side effects.

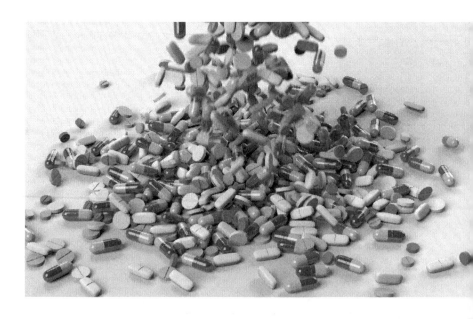

The average American consumes far too many prescription and over-the-counter drugs, often causing far worse medical problems than they are trying to solve.

The United States government has conducted an

unsuccessful war for decades against illegal drugs, but legal drugs kill far more people.

Follow the Golden Rule

This is not a religious but spiritual statement: The best way to avoid stress and anxiety is to follow the Golden Rule. The golden rule is the best recipe to achieve happiness, friendship, lasting love, and to evolve throughout one's life.

When we treat others with kindness, we launch positive waves across our species.

The norm is if a person treats us kind, we respond likewise.

Or, if a person mistreats us, we respond from hurt, anger, or frustration.

Break the norm! Be the person who treats others kind and sets a high bar for humanity.

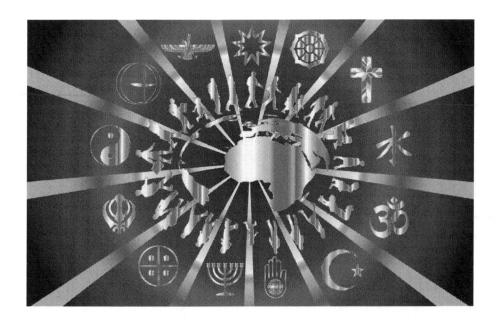

Follow the Golden Rule!

The world has too many preachers and not enough people following the Golden Rule. Follow the Golden Rule and use your live to make the world better.

Laugh when you can

Nothing fights depression, stress, and anxiety like laughter. When others give you reason to laugh, laugh. When they do not, search for the humor in every situation and make yourself laugh.

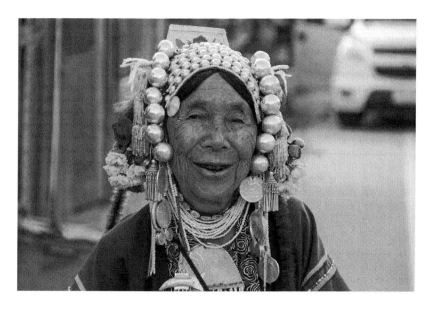

Laugh!

Make it a point to befriend people who make you laugh without hurting others.

Instead of seeing the worse in every situation; search for laughter like a comedian.

Spread laughter and you will be happier and healthier.

Avoid negativity

Negativity is the opposite of laughter, increasing stress, anxiety, and depression.

Two rules:

1. Avoid negative people.
2. Do not be a negative person.

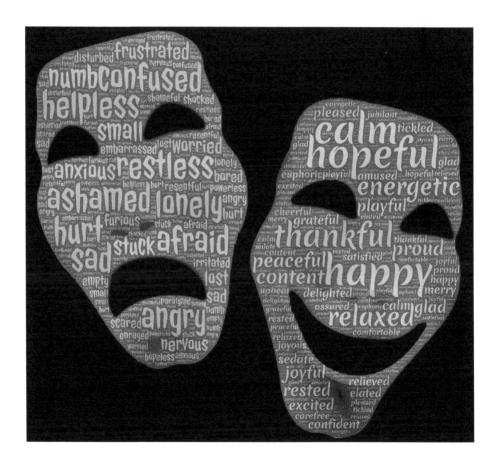

Manage cholesterol and blood pressure

In the chapters *Risk Factors, Symptoms, Diagnosis,* and *Stages,* we showed that high cholesterol and high blood pressure increase the risk of dementia.

High Cholesterol

Unhealthy eating habits causes most people's high cholesterol.

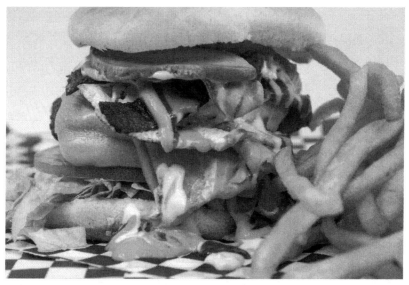

Not the meal of champions!

Eat food high in good cholesterol (HDL) and avoid bad cholesterol (LDL) to avoid or cure high cholesterol.

HDL (good) cholesterol absorbs HDL (bad) cholesterol and transport it to the liver, which will dispose of it[138].

Let's list some LDL and HDL foods, starting with the bad list.

Foods high in LDL (bad) cholesterol

- Dairy
- Trans fats

Foods high in HDL (good) cholesterol

- Beans and legumes
- Whole grains
- Fresh fruit
- Olive oil
- Avocados
- Tempeh
- Unfried Salmon (wild caught fatty fish)
- Red wine (Only 1 for women or 2 for men)
- Flax or Chia seeds
- Nuts

High Blood Pressure

Most people can avoid or fix blood pressure without medication. Not that you should stop taking medication your doctor prescribed, but high blood pressure is another medical condition a healthy lifestyle can avoid or fix. Work out a plan with your doctor.

Most get high blood pressure because we do not eat right, do not exercise, carry unhealthy body fat (the worst being abdominal fat), and otherwise do not take care of ourselves.

If we feed automobiles the wrong liquids in place of oil and gasoline, the infraction destroys the engine.

Why should it be different if we feed our bodies the wrong food?

Socialize

Positive social environments are healthy and reduce our risk of dementia.

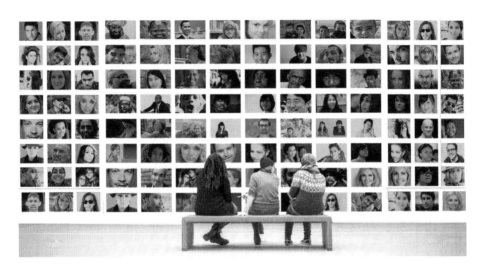

Do you engage regular socialization?

People who do not socialize increase their risk for the dementias whereas regular socializers decrease theirs.

By socialize, we do not mean hang out with people and drink yourself silly, do drugs, eat large portions of unhealthy food, or otherwise increase your risks of all diseases.

Engage in positive social functions:

- Become a community volunteer (also good for the soul)

- If you play a musical instrument, teach a few students
- If you do not play a musical instrument, take lessons
- Take a community college class or two
- Join an arts and crafts club
- Take art lessons and develop skills you can use every day
- Join a walking, jogging, swimming, or other club.
- Find several partners and play chess daily
- Invite friends over for a weekly card game
- Walk the neighborhood and be neighborly
- Join a bowling team
- Join a book reading club!
- Host a weekly dinner
- Organize picnics
- Join an astronomy club and study the stars
- Take a dancing class
- Coach or help coach kids (does not matter what sport)
- Constant visits to the local library (still a treasure!)

There are many regular social environments that inspire laughter, creativity, friendship, and a connectivity healthy humans require.

View your local options and pick the social engagements matching your likes and become a regular contributing member. Be the person you want those around you to be!

Review

Dementia is a deadly medical problem that modern science has no cure. Diagnosing the various pathologies is difficult, and general practitioners may or may not be qualified to make the call.

If you have the right doctor, include them in any major health decision. If you suspect you or a loved one might have dementia symptoms, request a neurologist or a specialist who specializes in dementia.

The best path to avoid the 16 primary dementias:

Chapter 8: CONCLUSION

Let's review what we covered.

You should now own a basic normal pressure hydrocephalus knowledge. You should understand normal pressure hydrocephalus:

- Definition
- Causes
- Diagnosis
- Stages
- Symptoms
- Risk factors
- Habits to be your healthiest, happiest, and most productive, and to possibly prevent or slow normal pressure hydrocephalus

Refer to chapters if you forget the fundamentals.

Updates

As science advances, so will this book. I update my health books at least once per year, so watch out for Amazon alerts.

THANK YOU FOR READING

Thank you for reading the entire book. While this is not a literary work to enjoy, I hope you gained useful knowledge of normal pressure hydrocephalus.

If this book benefitted you, please take a moment to share your thoughts in a review. Reader reviews help sell more books and keep producing more!

2019 Normal Pressure Hydrocephalus Book Review link =

https://amzn.to/2HfU1Tg

Look for annual updates to my health books. I follow new studies and will add any helpful information. Health and fitness are top priorities.

I hope you'll develop the habits suggested in this book. Good luck on your health journey. Live long and prosper, my friend.

All the best,

Jerry Beller & Beller Health

THE END

Of

2019 NORMAL PRESSURE HYDROCEPHALUS

Please continue for more information and books by Beller Health.

OTHER BELLER HEALTH BOOKS

Dementia Risk Factors, Symptoms, Diagnosis, Stages, Treatment, Prevention, Prevention

Alzheimer's Risk Factors & Symptoms

Behavioral Variant Frontotemporal Dementia (bvFTD)

Primary Progressive Aphasia (PPA)

Dementia with Lewy Bodies

Parkinson's disease

Huntington's Disease

Normal Pressure Hydrocephalus

Wernicke-Korsakoff Syndrome

LATE (Limbic-predominant age-related TDP-43 encephalopathy)

ALZHEIMER'S DEMENTIA SERIES

What is Alzheimer's? (2019), book 1

Alzheimer's Risk Factors (2019), book 2

Alzheimer's Symptoms (2019), book 3

Alzheimer's Diagnosis (2019), book 4

Alzheimer's Stages (2019), book 5

How to Prevent & Slow Alzheimer's (2019), book 6

Alzheimer's Treatment (2019), book 7

Other Beller Health Books

Be the Best You!

Dementia Types, Risk Factors, & Symptoms

Alzheimer's Collections

Vascular Dementia (2019)

Lewy Body Dementia (2019)

Frontotemporal Dementia (FTD)

You can view or purchase all Beller Health Books on Amazon at the following web address:

https://amzn.to/2TpDr8e

ABOUT THE AUTHOR

Beller Health is a team of health researchers and advocates who focus on diseases and cures. Veteran author and researcher Jerry Beller writes concise and well-documented medical books in everyday language.

Visit us at:

https://bellerhealth.com

1 'Hydro- | Definition of Hydro- in English by Oxford Dictionaries', *Oxford Dictionaries | English* <https://en.oxforddictionaries.com/definition/hydro-> [accessed 9 May 2019].

2 '-Cephalus', *TheFreeDictionary.Com* <https://medical-dictionary.thefreedictionary.com/-cephalus> [accessed 9 May 2019].

3 'Hydrocephalus | Genetic and Rare Diseases Information Center (GARD) – an NCATS Program' <https://rarediseases.info.nih.gov/diseases/6682/hydrocephalus> [accessed 18 February 2018].

4 'Normal Pressure Hydrocephalus | Hydrocephalus Association' <https://www.hydroassoc.org/normal-pressure-hydrocephalus/> [accessed 18 February 2018].

5 'Normal Pressure Hydrocephalus (NPH)', *Cleveland Clinic* <https://my.clevelandclinic.org/health/diseases/15849-normal-pressure-hydrocephalus-nph> [accessed 10 May 2019].

6 'Normal Pressure Hydrocephalus (NPH)', *Cleveland Clinic* <https://my.clevelandclinic.org/health/diseases/15849-normal-pressure-hydrocephalus-nph> [accessed 9 May 2019].

7 'Hydrocephalus Fact Sheet | National Institute of Neurological Disorders and Stroke' <https://www.ninds.nih.gov/Disorders/Patient-Caregiver-Education/Fact-Sheets/Hydrocephalus-Fact-Sheet> [accessed 9 May 2019].

8 Caren McHenry Martin, 'The "Reversible" Dementia of Idiopathic Normal Pressure Hydrocephalus', *The Consultant Pharmacist: The Journal of the American Society of Consultant Pharmacists*, 21.11 (2006), 888–92, 901–3.

9 'Facts and Stats', *Hydrocephalus Association* <https://www.hydroassoc.org/about-us/newsroom/facts-and-stats-2/> [accessed 10 May 2019].

10 'Normal Pressure Hydrocephalus (NPH) | AdventHealth

Neuroscience Institute'
<http://www.adventhealthneuroinstitute.com/programs/normal-pressure-hydrocephalus> [accessed 10 May 2019].

[11] 'Causes', *Hydrocephalus Association*
<https://www.hydroassoc.org/causes/> [accessed 10 May 2019].

[12] 'Home', *Alzheimer's Disease and Dementia* <https://alz.org/> [accessed 9 May 2019].

[13] 'Normal Pressure Hydrocephalus', *Alzheimer's Disease and Dementia* <https://alz.org/alzheimers-dementia/what-is-dementia/types-of-dementia/normal-pressure-hydrocephalus> [accessed 9 May 2019].

[14] 'Hydrocephalus Association', *Hydrocephalus Association* <https://www.hydroassoc.org/> [accessed 9 May 2019].

[15] 'Normal Pressure Hydrocephalus', *Hydrocephalus Association* <https://www.hydroassoc.org/normal-pressure-hydrocephalus/> [accessed 9 May 2019].

[16] Benito Pereira Damasceno, 'Neuroimaging in Normal Pressure Hydrocephalus', *Dementia & Neuropsychologia*, 9.4 (2015), 350–55 <https://doi.org/10.1590/1980-57642015DN94000350>.

[17] 'Clinical Examination - an Overview | ScienceDirect Topics' <https://www.sciencedirect.com/topics/medicine-and-dentistry/clinical-examination> [accessed 10 May 2019].

[18] Nir Giladi, Fay B Horak, and Jeffrey M. Hausdorff, 'Classification of Gait Disturbances: Distinguishing between Continuous and Episodic Changes', *Movement Disorders : Official Journal of the Movement Disorder Society*, 28.11 (2013) <https://doi.org/10.1002/mds.25672>.

[19] 'What Is Urinary Incontinence? - Urology Care Foundation' <https://www.urologyhealth.org/urologic-conditions/urinary-incontinence> [accessed 10 May 2019].

[20] 'Cognitive Impairment: A Call for Action, Now!', 4.

[21] 'Types of Brain Imaging Techniques'

<https://psychcentral.com/lib/types-of-brain-imaging-techniques/> [accessed 10 May 2019].

[22] 'CT Scan - Mayo Clinic' <https://www.mayoclinic.org/tests-procedures/ct-scan/about/pac-20393675> [accessed 10 May 2019].

[23] 'MRI Exam: How to Prepare & What to Expect | UCSF Radiology' <https://radiology.ucsf.edu/patient-care/prepare/mri> [accessed 10 May 2019].

[24] M. Venkatesh, 'Evans' Index | Radiology Reference Article | Radiopaedia.Org', *Radiopaedia* <https://radiopaedia.org/articles/evans-index-1?lang=us> [accessed 10 May 2019].

[25] Sara Kieffer, 'Cerebrospinal Fluid (CSF) Leak: Johns Hopkins Skull Base Tumor Center' <https://www.hopkinsmedicine.org/neurology_neurosurgery/centers_clinics/brain_tumor/center/skull-base/types/csf-leak.html> [accessed 10 May 2019].

[26] Ian K. Pople, 'Hydrocephalus and Shunts: What the Neurologist Should Know', *Journal of Neurology, Neurosurgery & Psychiatry*, 73.suppl 1 (2002), i17–22 <https://doi.org/10.1136/jnnp.73.suppl_1.i17>.

[27] Venessa L. Pinto, Prasanna Tadi, and Adebayo Adeyinka, 'Increased Intracranial Pressure', in *StatPearls* (Treasure Island (FL): StatPearls Publishing, 2019) <http://www.ncbi.nlm.nih.gov/books/NBK482119/> [accessed 10 May 2019].

[28] 'Normal Pressure Hydrocephalus', *Alzheimer's Disease and Dementia* <https://alz.org/alzheimers-dementia/what-is-dementia/types-of-dementia/normal-pressure-hydrocephalus> [accessed 10 May 2019].

[29] 'Normal Pressure Hydrocephalus (NPH) Diagnosis and Tests', *Cleveland Clinic* <https://my.clevelandclinic.org/health/diseases/15849-normal-pressure-hydrocephalus-nph/diagnosis-and-tests> [accessed 9 May 2019].

[30] Gagandeep Singh, 'Normal Pressure Hydrocephalus | Radiology Reference Article | Radiopaedia.Org', *Radiopaedia* <https://radiopaedia.org/articles/normal-pressure-

hydrocephalus?lang=us> [accessed 10 May 2019].

[31] 'Gait Analysis - an Overview | ScienceDirect Topics' <https://www.sciencedirect.com/topics/neuroscience/gait-analysis> [accessed 10 May 2019].

[32] Alvaro Muro-de-la-Herran, Begonya Garcia-Zapirain, and Amaia Mendez-Zorrilla, 'Gait Analysis Methods: An Overview of Wearable and Non-Wearable Systems, Highlighting Clinical Applications', *Sensors (Basel, Switzerland)*, 14.2 (2014), 3362–94 <https://doi.org/10.3390/s140203362>.

[33] 'Running Tech: What Is A Gait Analysis And Why Should Every Runner Have One?' <https://www.forbes.com/sites/leebelltech/2018/09/30/running-tech-what-is-a-gait-analysis-and-why-should-every-runner-have-one/#6a0f1fcf79bf> [accessed 10 May 2019].

[34] 'Gait Analysis | School of Podiatric Medicine' <https://podiatry.temple.edu/research/gait-study-center/gait-analysis> [accessed 10 May 2019].

[35] 'Medical Device Solutions - Gait Lab' <http://mds.clevelandclinic.org/Services/Gait-Lab.aspx> [accessed 10 May 2019].

[36] 'Normal Pressure Hydrocephalus', *Johns Hopkins Medicine Health Library* <https://www.hopkinsmedicine.org/health/conditions-and-diseases/hydrocephalus/normal-pressure-hydrocephalus> [accessed 10 May 2019].

[37] Imed Bouchrika and Mark S. Nixon, *Model-Based Feature Extraction for Gait Analysis and Recognition*.

[38] Imed Bouchrika and Mark S. Nixon, 'Model-Based Feature Extraction for Gait Analysis and Recognition', in *Proceedings of the 3rd International Conference on Computer Vision/Computer Graphics Collaboration Techniques*, MIRAGE'07 (Berlin, Heidelberg: Springer-Verlag, 2007), pp. 150–160 <http://dl.acm.org/citation.cfm?id=1759437.1759452> [accessed 10 May 2019].

[39] J. Bae, 'Gait Analysis Based on a Hidden Markov Model', in *2012 12th International Conference on Control, Automation and Systems*, 2012, pp. 1025–29.

[40] Ju Han and Bir Bhanu, 'Individual Recognition Using Gait Energy Image', *IEEE Transactions on Pattern Analysis and Machine Intelligence*, 28.2 (2006), 316–22 <https://doi.org/10.1109/TPAMI.2006.38>.

[41] Ju Han and Bir Bhanu, 'Individual Recognition Using Gait Energy Image', *IEEE Transactions on Pattern Analysis and Machine Intelligence*, 28 (2006), 316–22 <https://doi.org/10.1109/TPAMI.2006.38>.

[42] 'Cerebrospinal Fluid' <http://neuropathology-web.org/chapter14/chapter14CSF.html> [accessed 10 May 2019].

[43] 'Cerebral Spinal Fluid (CSF) Collection: MedlinePlus Medical Encyclopedia' <https://medlineplus.gov/ency/article/003428.htm> [accessed 11 May 2019].

[44] 'Diagnosing Normal Pressure Hydrocephalus' <https://nyulangone.org/conditions/normal-pressure-hydrocephalus-in-adults/diagnosis> [accessed 11 May 2019].

[45] E. E. Devito and others, 'The Neuropsychology of Normal Pressure Hydrocephalus (NPH)', *British Journal of Neurosurgery*, 19.3 (2005), 217–24 <https://doi.org/10.1080/02688690500201838>.

[46] 'NPH Left Untreated', *Hydrocephalus Association* <https://www.hydroassoc.org/nph-left-untreated/> [accessed 11 May 2019].

[47] 'New Insights into Normal Pressure Hydrocephalus', *Hydrocephalus Association* <https://www.hydroassoc.org/new-insights-into-normal-pressure-hydrocephalus/> [accessed 9 May 2019].

[48] 'Introducing the Pacific Adult Hydrocephalus Center', *Pacific Neuroscience Institute*, 2016 <https://www.pacificneuroscienceinstitute.org/blog/hydrocephalus-related-conditions/introducing-pacific-adult-hydrocephalus-center/> [accessed 10 May 2019].

[49] 'Brain Matters: Dementia Caused By Normal Pressure Hydrocephalus Can Be Reversible', *Pacific Neuroscience Institute*, 2019 <https://www.pacificneuroscienceinstitute.org/blog/hydrocephalus/brain-matters-dementia-caused-by-normal-pressure-hydrocephalus-can-be-reversible/> [accessed 10 May 2019].

[50] 'Diagnosing Normal Pressure Hydrocephalus | Swedish Medical Center Seattle and Issaquah' <https://www.swedish.org:443/services/neuroscience-institute/our-services/hydrocephalus/normal-pressure-hydrocephalus/diagnosing-normal-pressure-hydrocephalus> [accessed 10 May 2019].

[51] Radiological Society of North America (RSNA) and American College of Radiology (ACR), 'Lumbar Puncture (Spinal Tap)' <https://www.radiologyinfo.org/en/info.cfm?pg=spinaltap> [accessed 10 May 2019].

[52] 'Lumbar Puncture | Johns Hopkins Medicine' <https://www.hopkinsmedicine.org/health/treatment-tests-and-therapies/lumbar-puncture> [accessed 10 May 2019].

[53] National Center for Biotechnology Information and others, *What Happens during a Lumbar Puncture (Spinal Tap)?* (Institute for Quality and Efficiency in Health Care (IQWiG), 2016) <https://www.ncbi.nlm.nih.gov/books/NBK367574/> [accessed 10 May 2019].

[54] 'Lumbar Puncture (Spinal Tap) - Mayo Clinic' <https://www.mayoclinic.org/tests-procedures/lumbar-puncture/about/pac-20394631> [accessed 10 May 2019].

[55] 'About Your Ventriculoperitoneal (VP) Shunt Surgery', *Memorial Sloan Kettering Cancer Center* <https://www.mskcc.org/cancer-care/patient-education/about-your-ventriculoperitoneal-vp-shunt-surgery> [accessed 10 May 2019].

[56] 'Ventriculoperitonial Shunt', *Pacific Adult Hydrocephalus Center* <https://www.pacificneuroscienceinstitute.org/hydrocephalus/treatment/shunt-procedures/ventriculoperitoneal-shunt/> [accessed 10 May 2019].

57 'Shunt Systems', *Hydrocephalus Association* <https://www.hydroassoc.org/shunt-systems/> [accessed 10 May 2019].

58 Julia Cannon, 'Shunt Procedure | Johns Hopkins Medicine in Baltimore, MD' <https://www.hopkinsmedicine.org/neurology_neurosurgery/centers_clinics/cerebral-fluid/procedures/shunts.html> [accessed 10 May 2019].

59 Julia Cannon, 'Shunt Procedure | Johns Hopkins Medicine in Baltimore, MD' <https://www.hopkinsmedicine.org/neurology_neurosurgery/centers_clinics/cerebral-fluid/procedures/shunts.html> [accessed 10 May 2019].

60 Hiroaki Kazui, '[Cognitive impairment in patients with idiopathic normal pressure hydrocephalus]', *Brain and Nerve = Shinkei Kenkyu No Shinpo*, 60.3 (2008), 225–31.

61 A. Berardelli and others, 'Pathophysiology of Bradykinesia in Parkinson's Disease', *Brain: A Journal of Neurology*, 124.Pt 11 (2001), 2131–46.

62 'Cognitive Therapy for NPH Patients | Hydrocephalus Association' <https://www.hydroassoc.org/cognitive-therapy-for-nph-patients/> [accessed 18 February 2018].

63 'AANS | Adult-Onset Hydrocephalus' <http://www.aans.org/Patients/Neurosurgical-Conditions-and-Treatments/Adult-Onset-Hydrocephalus> [accessed 18 February 2018].

64 'Hydrocephalus > Condition at Yale Medicine', *Yale Medicine* <https://www.yalemedicine.org/conditions/hydrocephalus/> [accessed 18 February 2018].

65 'Normal Pressure Hydrocephalus: Practice Essentials, Background, Pathophysiology', 2019 <https://emedicine.medscape.com/article/1150924-overview> [accessed 10 May 2019].

[66] 'Symptoms and Diagnosis | Hydrocephalus Association' <https://www.hydroassoc.org/symptoms-and-diagnosis-nph/> [accessed 18 February 2018].

[67] 'Normal Pressure Hydrocephalus - an Overview | ScienceDirect Topics' <https://www.sciencedirect.com/topics/neuroscience/normal-pressure-hydrocephalus> [accessed 18 February 2018].

[68] 'SHYMA.Pdf' <http://www.hydroassoc.org/docs/SHYMA.pdf> [accessed 18 February 2018].

[69] 'Hydrocephalus – Causes, Symptom and Surgical Treatments' <https://www.aans.org/> [accessed 10 May 2019].

[70] 'Hydrocephalus (for Parents) - KidsHealth' <https://kidshealth.org/en/parents/hydrocephalus.html> [accessed 10 May 2019].

[71] 'Normal Pressure Hydrocephalus', *Child Neurology Foundation* <https://www.childneurologyfoundation.org/disorder/normal-pressure-hydrocephalus/> [accessed 10 May 2019].

[72] Harvard Health Publishing, 'Hydrocephalus', *Harvard Health* <https://www.health.harvard.edu/a_to_z/hydrocephalus-a-to-z> [accessed 10 May 2019].

[73] 'Hydrocephalus', *NORD (National Organization for Rare Disorders)* <https://rarediseases.org/rare-diseases/hydrocephalus/> [accessed 10 May 2019].

[74] 'Normal Pressure Hydrocephalus'.

[75] 'Hydrocephalus'.

[76] 'Normal Pressure Hydrocephalus (NPH) | Signs, Symptoms, & Diagnosis', *Dementia* <//www.alz.org/dementia/normal-pressure-hydrocephalus-nph.asp> [accessed 18 February 2018].

[77] 'Normal Pressure Hydrocephalus'.

[78] 'Hydrocephalus Fact Sheet | National Institute of Neurological Disorders and Stroke' <https://www.ninds.nih.gov/Disorders/Patient-Caregiver-Education/Fact-Sheets/Hydrocephalus-Fact-Sheet> [accessed 18 February 2018].

[79] 'Hydrocephalus Clinical Presentation: History, Physical, Causes' <https://emedicine.medscape.com/article/1135286-clinical> [accessed 11 May 2019].

[80] 'Hydrocephalus - Symptoms and Causes - Mayo Clinic' <https://www.mayoclinic.org/diseases-conditions/hydrocephalus/symptoms-causes/syc-20373604> [accessed 11 May 2019].

[81] Krauss Joachim K. and others, 'Vascular Risk Factors and Arteriosclerotic Disease in Idiopathic Normal-Pressure Hydrocephalus of the Elderly', *Stroke*, 27.1 (1996), 24–29 <https://doi.org/10.1161/01.STR.27.1.24>.

[82] 'Normal Pressure Hydrocephalus Information Page | National Institute of Neurological Disorders and Stroke' <https://www.ninds.nih.gov/Disorders/All-Disorders/Normal-Pressure-Hydrocephalus-Information-Page> [accessed 18 February 2018].

[83] 'Normal Pressure Hydrocephalus' <http://www.mayfieldclinic.com/pe-NPH.htm> [accessed 18 February 2018].

[84] 'Role of Diet and Nutritional Supplements in Parkinson's Disease Progression' <https://www.hindawi.com/journals/omcl/2017/6405278/> [accessed 24 April 2019].

[85] 'Fitness Fitness Basics', *Mayo Clinic* <https://www.mayoclinic.org/healthy-lifestyle/fitness/basics/fitness-basics/hlv-20049447> [accessed 7 May 2019].

[86] 'Physical Activity for a Healthy Weight | Healthy Weight | CDC', 2019

<https://www.cdc.gov/healthyweight/physical_activity/index.html> [accessed 7 May 2019].

[87] Fitness & Nutrition President's Council on Sports, 'Physical Activity Guidelines for Americans', *HHS.Gov*, 2012 <https://www.hhs.gov/fitness/be-active/physical-activity-guidelines-for-americans/index.html> [accessed 7 May 2019].

[88] D. E. Warburton, N. Gledhill, and A. Quinney, 'Musculoskeletal Fitness and Health', *Canadian Journal of Applied Physiology = Revue Canadienne De Physiologie Appliquee*, 26.2 (2001), 217–37.

[89] M. Harold Laughlin, 'Joseph B. Wolfe Memorial Lecture. Physical Activity in Prevention and Treatment of Coronary Disease: The Battle Line Is in Exercise Vascular Cell Biology', *Medicine and Science in Sports and Exercise*, 36.3 (2004), 352–62.

[90] Isabel Ferreira and others, 'Longitudinal Changes in .VO2max: Associations with Carotid IMT and Arterial Stiffness', *Medicine and Science in Sports and Exercise*, 35.10 (2003), 1670–78 <https://doi.org/10.1249/01.MSS.0000089247.37563.4B>.

[91] Andrew Maiorana and others, 'Exercise and the Nitric Oxide Vasodilator System', *Sports Medicine (Auckland, N.Z.)*, 33.14 (2003), 1013–35 <https://doi.org/10.2165/00007256-200333140-00001>.

[92] James A. Mortimer and Yaakov Stern, 'Physical Exercise and Activity May Be Important in Reducing Dementia Risk at Any Age', *Neurology*, 92.8 (2019), 362–63 <https://doi.org/10.1212/WNL.0000000000006935>.

[93] Zi Zhou and others, 'Association between Exercise and the Risk of Dementia: Results from a Nationwide Longitudinal Study in China', *BMJ Open*, 7.12 (2017), e017497 <https://doi.org/10.1136/bmjopen-2017-017497>.

[94] Helena Hörder and others, 'Author Response: Midlife Cardiovascular Fitness and Dementia: A 44-Year Longitudinal Population Study in Women', *Neurology*, 91.16 (2018), 763–763 <https://doi.org/10.1212/WNL.0000000000006350>.

[95] Jacqueline Howard CNN, 'Your Dementia Risk Tied to How Fit

You Are', *CNN* <https://www.cnn.com/2018/03/14/health/dementia-risk-fitness-study/index.html> [accessed 8 May 2019].

[96] Sam Norton and others, 'Potential for Primary Prevention of Alzheimer's Disease: An Analysis of Population-Based Data', *The Lancet Neurology*, 13.8 (2014), 788–94 <https://doi.org/10.1016/S1474-4422(14)70136-X>.

[97] 'Executive Summary: Physical Activity Guidelines for Americans, 2nd Edition', 7.

[98] Eric B. Larson and others, 'Exercise Is Associated with Reduced Risk for Incident Dementia among Persons 65 Years of Age and Older', *Annals of Internal Medicine*, 144.2 (2006), 73–81.

[99] Susan Mayor, 'Regular Exercise Reduces Risk of Dementia and Alzheimer's Disease', *BMJ : British Medical Journal*, 332.7534 (2006), 137 <https://www.ncbi.nlm.nih.gov/pmc/articles/PMC1336790/> [accessed 7 May 2019].

[100] 'What Is the DASH Diet?' <http://dashdiet.org/what-is-the-dash-diet.html> [accessed 7 May 2019].

[101] 'Alzheimer's Prevention Clinic | Weill Cornell Medicine' <https://weillcornell.org/services/neurology/alzheimers-disease-memory-disorders-program/our-services/alzheimers-prevention-clinic> [accessed 7 May 2019].

[102] 'Patient Care | Weill Cornell Medicine' <https://weillcornell.org/> [accessed 7 May 2019].

[103] Paul T. Williams, 'Lower Risk of Alzheimer's Disease Mortality with Exercise, Statin, and Fruit Intake', *Journal of Alzheimer's Disease*, 44.4 (2015), 1121–29 <https://doi.org/10.3233/JAD-141929>.

[104] 'Robert C. Green, MD, MPH - Department of Medicine' <http://researchfaculty.brighamandwomens.org/BRIProfile.aspx?id=5921> [accessed 8 May 2019].

[105] Robert C. Green and others, 'Depression as a Risk Factor for Alzheimer Disease: The MIRAGE Study', *Archives of Neurology*, 60.5 (2003), 753–59 <https://doi.org/10.1001/archneur.60.5.753>.

[106] Vonetta M. Dotson, May A. Beydoun, and Alan B. Zonderman,

'Recurrent Depressive Symptoms and the Incidence of Dementia and Mild Cognitive Impairment', *Neurology*, 75.1 (2010), 27–34 <https://doi.org/10.1212/WNL.0b013e3181e62124>.

[107] Kaarin J. Anstey and others, 'Smoking as a Risk Factor for Dementia and Cognitive Decline: A Meta-Analysis of Prospective Studies', *American Journal of Epidemiology*, 166.4 (2007), 367–78 <https://doi.org/10.1093/aje/kwm116>.

[108] Minna Rusanen and others, 'Heavy Smoking in Midlife and Long-Term Risk of Alzheimer Disease and Vascular Dementia', *Archives of Internal Medicine*, 171.4 (2011), 333–39 <https://doi.org/10.1001/archinternmed.2010.393>.

[109] 'Tobacco Facts | State of Tobacco Control', *American Lung Association* <https://www.lung.org/our-initiatives/tobacco/reports-resources/sotc/facts.html> [accessed 8 May 2019].

[110] CDCTobaccoFree, 'Fast Facts', *Centers for Disease Control and Prevention*, 2019 <https://www.cdc.gov/tobacco/data_statistics/fact_sheets/fast_facts/index.htm> [accessed 8 May 2019].

[111] 'WHO | WHO Report on the Global Tobacco Epidemic 2017', *WHO* <http://www.who.int/tobacco/global_report/2017/en/> [accessed 8 May 2019].

[112] Prabhat Jha and others, '21st-Century Hazards of Smoking and Benefits of Cessation in the United States', *New England Journal of Medicine*, 368.4 (2013), 341–50 <https://doi.org/10.1056/NEJMsa1211128>.

[113] 'Ftc_cigarette_report_2017.Pdf' <https://www.ftc.gov/system/files/documents/reports/federal-trade-commission-cigarette-report-2017-federal-trade-commission-smokeless-tobacco-report/ftc_cigarette_report_2017.pdf> [accessed 8 May 2019].

[114] P. A. Wolf and others, 'Cigarette Smoking as a Risk Factor for Stroke. The Framingham Study', *JAMA*, 259.7 (1988), 1025–29.

[115] John A Ambrose and Rajat S Barua, 'The Pathophysiology of Cigarette Smoking and Cardiovascular Disease: An Update', *Journal of*

the *American College of Cardiology*, 43.10 (2004), 1731–37
<https://doi.org/10.1016/j.jacc.2003.12.047>.

[116] Brian L. Rostron, Cindy M. Chang, and Terry F. Pechacek, 'Estimation of Cigarette Smoking-Attributable Morbidity in the United States', *JAMA Internal Medicine*, 174.12 (2014), 1922–28 <https://doi.org/10.1001/jamainternmed.2014.5219>.

[117] 'American Psychological Association (APA)', *Https://Www.Apa.Org* <https://www.apa.org/index> [accessed 8 May 2019].

[118] 'Anxiety', *Https://Www.Apa.Org* <https://www.apa.org/topics/anxiety/index> [accessed 8 May 2019].

[119] Olivia I. Okereke and others, 'High Phobic Anxiety Is Related to Lower Leukocyte Telomere Length in Women', *PLOS ONE*, 7.7 (2012), e40516 <https://doi.org/10.1371/journal.pone.0040516>.

[120] 'Lifestyle Changes May Lengthen Telomeres, A Measure of Cell Aging | UC San Francisco', *Lifestyle Changes May Lengthen Telomeres, A Measure of Cell Aging | UC San Francisco* <https://www.ucsf.edu/news/2013/09/108886/lifestyle-changes-may-lengthen-telomeres-measure-cell-aging> [accessed 8 May 2019].

[121] Michael T. Lee focus97, 'Preventive Medicine Research Institute', *Preventive Medicine Research Institute* <http://www.pmri.org> [accessed 8 May 2019].

[122] 'Lifestyle Changes May Lengthen Telomeres, A Measure of Cell Aging | UC San Francisco'.

[123] 'Lifestyle Changes May Lengthen Telomeres, A Measure of Cell Aging | UC San Francisco'.

[124] 'American Psychological Association (APA)'.

[125] Linda Mah, Malcolm A. Binns, and David C. Steffens, 'Anxiety Symptoms in Amnestic Mild Cognitive Impairment Are Associated with Medial Temporal Atrophy and Predict Conversion to Alzheimer Disease', *The American Journal of Geriatric Psychiatry*, 23.5 (2015), 466–76 <https://doi.org/10.1016/j.jagp.2014.10.005>.

[126] 'Frontiers in Neuroscience'

<https://www.frontiersin.org/journals/neuroscience> [accessed 8 May 2019].

[127] Marion Mortamais and others, 'Anxiety and 10-Year Risk of Incident Dementia—An Association Shaped by Depressive Symptoms: Results of the Prospective Three-City Study', *Frontiers in Neuroscience*, 12 (2018) <https://doi.org/10.3389/fnins.2018.00248>.

[128] 'JAMA Network | Home of JAMA and the Specialty Journals of the American Medical Association' <https://jamanetwork.com/> [accessed 8 May 2019].

[129] 'Robert Pietrzak, PhD, MPH > Psychiatry | Yale School of Medicine' <https://medicine.yale.edu/psychiatry/people/robert_pietrzak-2.profile> [accessed 8 May 2019].

[130] 'Clinical Neurosciences PTSD Research Program > Psychiatry | Yale School of Medicine' <https://medicine.yale.edu/psychiatry/research/programs/clinical_people/ptsd.aspx> [accessed 8 May 2019].

[131] Amy Gimson and others, 'Support for Midlife Anxiety Diagnosis as an Independent Risk Factor for Dementia: A Systematic Review', *BMJ Open*, 8.4 (2018), e019399 <https://doi.org/10.1136/bmjopen-2017-019399>.

[132] Harvard Health Publishing, 'Health Information and Medical Information', *Harvard Health* <https://www.health.harvard.edu/> [accessed 8 May 2019].

[133] Harvard Health Publishing, 'Two Types of Drugs You May Want to Avoid for the Sake of Your Brain', *Harvard Health* <https://www.health.harvard.edu/mind-and-mood/two-types-of-drugs-you-may-want-to-avoid-for-the-sake-of-your-brain> [accessed 8 May 2019].

[134] 'Home', *Nhs.Uk*, 2018 <https://www.nhs.uk/> [accessed 8 May 2019].

[135] 'Can Dementia Be Prevented?', *Nhs.Uk*, 2017 <https://www.nhs.uk/conditions/dementia/dementia-prevention/> [accessed 8 May 2019].

[136] Michaël Schwarzinger and others, 'Contribution of Alcohol Use Disorders to the Burden of Dementia in France 2008–13: A Nationwide Retrospective Cohort Study', *The Lancet Public Health*, 3.3 (2018), e124–32 <https://doi.org/10.1016/S2468-2667(18)30022-7>.

[137] Jürgen Rehm and others, 'Alcohol Use and Dementia: A Systematic Scoping Review', *Alzheimer's Research & Therapy*, 11.1 (2019), 1 <https://doi.org/10.1186/s13195-018-0453-0>.

[138] CDC, 'LDL and HDL Cholesterol: "Bad" and "Good" Cholesterol', *Centers for Disease Control and Prevention*, 2017 <https://www.cdc.gov/cholesterol/ldl_hdl.htm> [accessed 24 April 2019].

Made in the USA
Middletown, DE
31 July 2020